Table of Contents

Introduction

Understanding Lung cancer can be beneficial for those diagnosed, family or friends, and the community. Lung cancer is caused by many things —not just smoking. Understanding the signs, symptoms, treatment and prevention will better suit everyone.

In this guide to Lung Cancer you will learn about Lung Cancer, the human lung, treatment and prevention, as well as, coping and statistics.

This guide to Lung Cancer is made specifically as an instrument of knowledge and basic understanding.

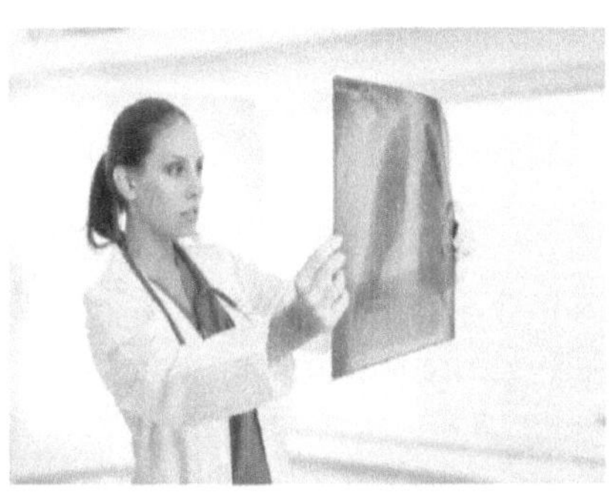

What is Lung Cancer?

Cancer is so prevalent that it is most likely you or someone you know has dealt with this condition is some capacity. Although there are many different types of cancer, lung cancer is one of the most common. Learning more about this type of cancer helps to spread awareness and allows for early detection.

What is Lung Cancer?

In basic terms, lung cancer is the uncontrolled growth of cells that are not normal within the lungs. These abnormal cells change the overall shape and function of the lungs. This is due to the fact that normal cells are designed and programmed to alter the shape and function in a specific way, but abnormal cells reproduce at a rapid rate and are not properly programmed. This leads to high production of cells that can result in tumors that further negatively affect the lung. This means that tumor growth can keep the lung from functioning at a high level.

What about Detecting Tumors?

Detecting tumor growth on the lung is not always easy. Lungs are large in size, which means that tumors can sometimes grow for years without being detected. This is due to the fact that lung cancer has the ability to spread outside the lungs and leave no signs or symptoms behind. It is also common for persistent coughs that are noticeable with lung cancer to be misdiagnosed as a cold or bronchitis. Early detection of cancer is not always normal.

Is This Type of Cancer Common?

Lung cancer is so common that it is one of the most common types of cancer in the entire United States. Almost 15% of all new cases of cancer diagnosed each year are attributed to lung cancer. This means that about 170,000 new cases of lung cancer pop up each year. A little more than half of the lung cancer cases are men, but research shows that women are being diagnosed with lung cancer at a higher rate than ever before. In fact, more women die of lung cancer than breast cancer.

Link to Smoking

Many of the cases that involve lung cancer can be linked to smoking. Even though the majority of the individuals that are diagnosed with lung cancer smoke cigarettes, not all people that smoke get lung cancer. It is also common that people diagnosed with lung cancer have never smoked before in their life. Smoking is not the only cause of this condition.

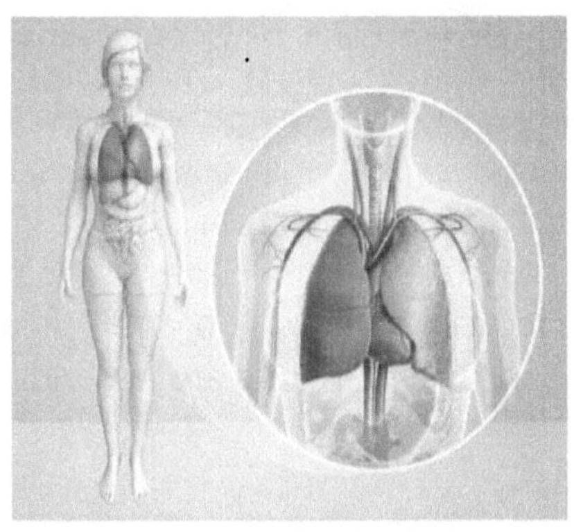

What is a Human Lung?

Have you ever tried to hold your breath for any significant period of time? If so, you will quickly realize how important lungs are in how your body functions as a whole. Human lungs are organs within the body that carry out the function of respiration. This means that the main job of the lungs is to remove oxygen from the atmosphere and allow it into the bloodstream. It is then ejected back out into the atmosphere again.

How Do They Work?

This vital role of taking oxygen from the atmosphere and putting it into your bloodstream is made possible through contracting and expanding. This role of contracting and expanding is supported by the diaphragm due to signals that are sent by the brain. The brain receives signals with the act of contracting and expanding needs to be sped up or slowed down. When you are running or exerting yourself through exercise or when you are sleeping, different signals are being sent from your brain to indicate the rate at which you should be contracting or expanding your lungs.

Think of it this way, when the diaphragm is contracting the lungs pull in a motion that is downward. This allows for their capacity to increase and extracts the air out. Once the diaphragm relaxes, all the oxygen that was not taken into the bloodstream is ejected from the lungs. In addition to the unabsorbed oxygen, carbon dioxide is also ejected from the lungs.

The entire function of human lungs is not solely to provide the body with oxygen-rich blood. This may be the main function and priority, but the human lungs do so much more within the body. Lungs actually act as a protective cushion for the heart. This is due to the fact that they almost completely surround the heart within your body. It should also be noted that the lymph nodes that surround your lungs are responsible for filtering germs and impurities from your system.

Humans Have Two Lungs

Humans have tow lungs and the left lung is divided into two lobes. The right lung is divided into three lobes and together, these two lungs have a normal surface area that is equivalent to one side of a tennis court. Common diseases of the lungs include pneumonia, asthma, and emphysema and lung cancer. These lung diseases have their own specific symptoms.

Signs and Symptoms of Lung Cancer

Lung cancer is one of the most common types of cancer in the entire United States. However, early detection of this disease is not always possible due to the lack of noticeable symptoms. Although survival rate is greatly impacted by early diagnosis. Many people with lung cancer experience tumor growth for years before they are properly diagnosed.

What is Lung Cancer?

Lung cancer is described as the growth of abnormal cells within the lungs. This allows for the fast reproduction of cells that are not properly programed with function and shape in mind. This allows for tumor growth as a result, but tumors growing on the lungs are not always detected early. Even though tumors keep your lungs from functioning at a high level, many of the symptoms of lung cancer either go unnoticed or are misdiagnosed.

Importance of Noticing Symptoms Early

Many types of lung cancer do not cause symptoms early on. This results in symptoms often not being noticed or diagnosed until the condition has spread to a point beyond curing. However, it is possible that if you go to your doctor at first sign of symptoms, you may get an early diagnosis. During the early stages of this cancer, almost all treatment options are much more effective.

Here are some of the most common lung cancer symptoms that you should be on the lookout for:

- A cough that worsens or persists over time
- Pain in the chest that worsens when you cough, breathe or laugh
- Hoarse voice
- Weight loss and the disappearance of your appetite
- Constant tiredness and weakness
- Frequent infections including bronchitis and pneumonia that persist

- Wheezing

If the early signs and symptoms of lung cancer are not noticed, it may spread to other organs and allow for a new set of signs and symptoms:

- Pain in your bones, most prevalent in hips and back
- Frequent headaches, dizziness and balance issues due to the spread of this cancer to your nervous system
- Yellow skin and eyes
- Noticeable lumps of the body near the neck and collarbone.

Many of the signs and symptoms that are common with lung cancer are hard to detect and can often be misdiagnosed. It is important to be aware of all signs and symptoms of this disease, so that you can detect it early on. Early detection of lung cancer is essential to survival rate.

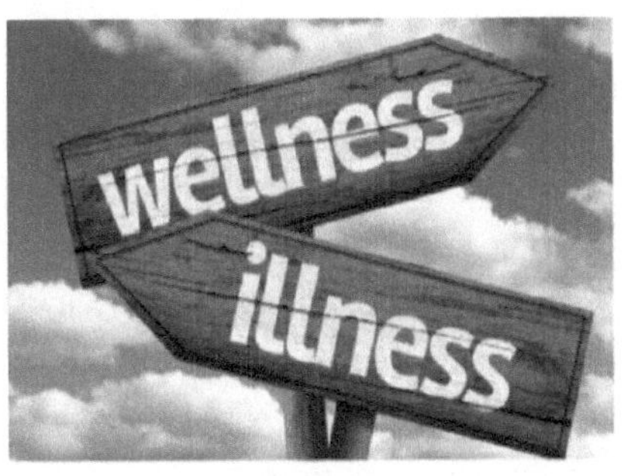

What Are Causes of Lung Cancer?

Lung cancer is one of the most common types of cancer in the United States and almost 15% of new cancer cases each year are attributed to this type. Lung cancer involves the growth and rapid production of abnormal cells within the lungs that negatively effects the function and shape. This results in tumor growth that can further disturb and inhibit the overall function of the lungs. Since lung cancer is so common, it is important to understand the causes that it can be linked to.

Smoking is the Most Common Cause

One of the most common causes of lung cancer can be attributed to smoking. Many of the substances that are found in tobacco are linked to cancer and are known carcinogens. This means that tobacco products are filled with cancer-causing ingredients. In many cases of lung cancer, it is these carcinogens that cause cell damage within the lungs. Once cells are damaged, it is normally only a period of time before cancer growth occurs.

Are All Smokers Diagnosed With Lung Cancer?

Even though smoking is found to be the most common cause of lung cancer, it is impossible to predict each smoker's risk of developing this form of cancer over time. The factors of smoking that have the most impact on the onset of lung cancer include the age when smoking began, the period of time that smoking has taken place and the number of cigarettes that are smoked daily. It is important to note that not every smoker gets lung cancer and not all individuals with lung cancer are smokers. This means that smoking is a main cause, but it is not the only cause of lung cancer.

Other Causes

Even though you may not smoke, being exposed to passive smoking can also cause lung cancer. Being exposed to asbestos or other cancer-causing agents at work can also lead to lung cancer. Radiation exposure and exposure to radon gas are also known causes. Individuals that smoke and exposed to these cancer causing agents increase their chances of lung cancer diagnosis by high rates.

Are You At Risk?

Some research on lung cancer causes has found that many individuals are simply more at risk for developing this type of cancer than others. These individuals are not able to deal with cancer-causing agents in their body and smoking only results in higher risk.

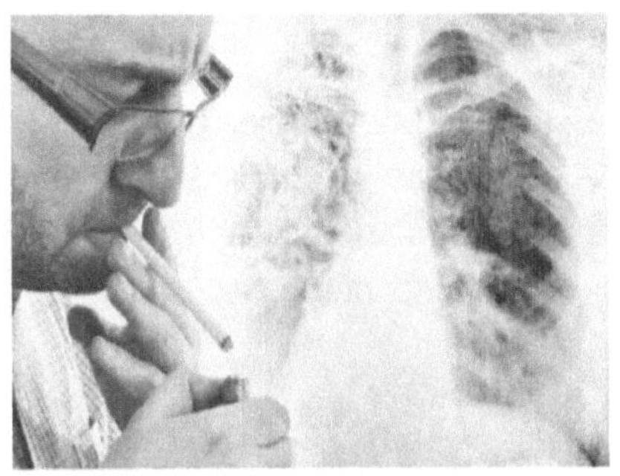

Lung Cancer and Smoking

Lung cancer can be attributed to a variety of different causes, but smoking seems to be the most common and the most prevalent. Lung cancer is a common type of cancer that accounts for about 15% of cancer cases each year, but early diagnosis is not always easy. The symptoms of this type of cancer can go undetected or are often misdiagnosed. This means that it is incredibly important to know about the risk factors that are associated with lung cancer. Smoking is the number one risk factor and can increase your chances of being diagnosed with this type of cancer substantially.

Smoking Risk Factor

The number one risk factor of lung cancer is smoking. It is a fact that more than 90% of lung cancers are caused by smoking. Other tobacco products including cigars and pipes also can be linked to the onset of lung cancer. Tobacco products are filled with carcinogens, which are cancer-causing agents. It is true that tobacco smoke contains more than 7,000 toxic chemicals, which are known to cause cancer.

How Much Do Your Chances Increase?

Individuals that smoke are between 16 and 31 times more likely to get lung cancer than those individuals that do not smoke. Simply smoking cigarettes a few times each week can increase your risk, but the more you smoke each day is linked to the likelihood that you will get lung cancer. How long you have smoked and the amount of cigarettes that you smoke daily are the factors that matter most.

What is You Quit?

Individuals the stop smoking lower the risk of lung cancer, but still have a higher chance of getting diagnosed than those people that never smoked before. No matter what age you are, lowering your chances of getting lung cancer by quitting smoking is possible.

Smoking and Cancer

Not only is smoking the number one cause of lung cancer, but it also can cause cancer in other areas of the body. Aside from the lungs, smoking can be attributed to cancer of the mouth, nose, throat, bladder, kidney, pancreas stomach, blood and much more.

Do You Have to Smoke to Get Lung Cancer?

What are the Diagnoses of Lung Cancer?

Lung cancer is gradual over time and not always diagnosed right away. It is caused by the growth of abnormal cells within the lungs that result in tumor growth. This impairs the shape and function of the lungs. Diagnosing lung cancer is not always easy in the beginning stages. However, early diagnosis of lung cancer is critical to the survival rate of this condition.

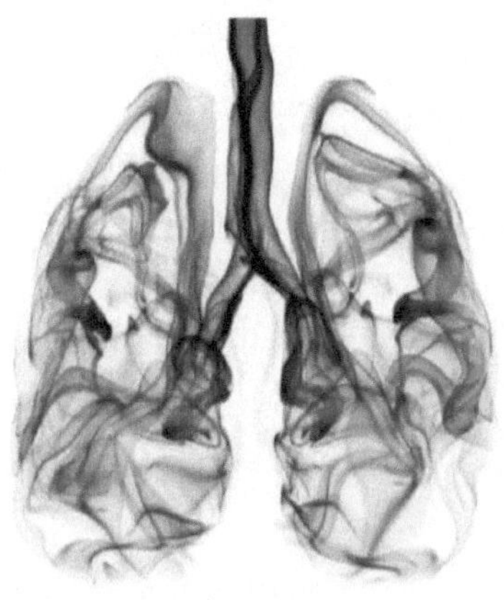

How Is Lung Cancer Diagnosed?

When you believe that you may be suffering from symptoms of lung cancer, your doctor can perform a routine exam that may provide some insight. If any of these are revealed during your exam, lung cancer might be suspected:

- Swollen lymph nodes
- Abdomen pain and growth
- Trouble breathing
- Sounds in the lungs that are not normal
- Dullness in chest
- Droopy eyelids
- Weakened arm
- Swelling of the face

If any of these early signs are noticed by your doctor, further testing will be done to see if you do have lung cancer. Many lung cancers result in blood levels that contain high amounts of hormones and certain substances. If no other cause for these blood levels can be found, lung cancer should be considered. It is possible for lung cancer to spread to other areas of the body. This means that it might first be found in these other regions, before it is evidenced within the lungs.

X-Ray Diagnosis

Once actual symptoms of lung cancer are noticed, it is possible to diagnose this cancer with an x-ray. In some cases, lung cancer that has not begun to cause symptoms can be spotted on an x-ray, but this is not common. A CT scan of your chest might sometimes show lung cancer even though no other symptoms are noticed. A detailed scan of eth chest will then be ordered to see if lung cancer does in fact exist.

Lung Biopsy

It is possible for the fluids within the lungs to reveal the presence of cancerous cells, but lung diagnosis is not usually conclusive until a lung biopsy is performed. This involves the patient being placed under light anesthesia. A doctor will then place a tube through the nose and into the air passage to the tumor. A tiny sample of eth tumor will be removed to confirm the presence of lung cancer. This is the type of lung cancer diagnosis that is the most accurate and conclusive.

Although smoking is the main cause of lung cancer, it is not the only cause. Smoking does not automatically mean you will get lung cancer. Many people that smoke never get lung cancer and many people that don't smoke are diagnosed. Smoking is simply a risk factor and is known to be the number one culprit of this cancer type.

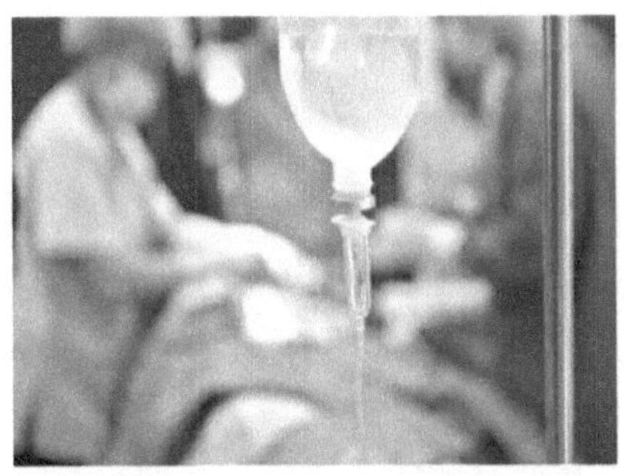

How is Lung Cancer Treated Using Surgery?

Lung cancer does not often have noticeable signs or symptoms in the early stages, which means that the cancerous tumor can grow for years before it is properly diagnosed. Survival rate is tied to time of diagnosis, but the treatment option for your cancer is also linked to when you are diagnosed.

What Factors go into the Treatment Option?

The treatment option that is best for treating your lung cancer depends on the type and extent of your condition. This means that before a doctor comes to you with an available treatment option, the type, size and location of the tumor need to be known. It is also important to know if the cancer has spread to any other region of the body.

Staging and Treatment Option

All of this information is essential, because it offers a staging analysis of the lung cancer. This staging is necessary because it allows for the best treatment option to be chosen. Staging allows for your doctor to better predict how your cancer will progress over time and the chances that it might return. Lower stages generally are linked to a better prognosis and a treatment option that is less severe.

How is Lung Cancer Staged?

Lung cancer is staged through biopsy and imaging. This means that chest and CT scans and a biopsy of the tumor on the lung must be performed before staging can be determined. Once the stage of lung cancer has been fully identified, it is easier to select the right treatment option.

Surgery is one of the types of treatment options that is available for individuals that are diagnosed with lung cancer. The type of stage you are diagnosed with determines the type of surgical procedure that will be identified as eth most appropriate. A wedge resection is a common surgical treatment for lung cancer and involves the removal of a small part of the lung where the growth is isolated. In some cases, a whole lobe of the lung can be moved if the growth is larger and this surgical procedure is known as a lobectomy.

What is a Pneumonectomy?

This is a more invasive surgical procedure that involves the removal of an entire lung. In contrast, a new and less invasive surgical treatment option for lung cancer that is becoming more popular is known as video assisted thoracic surgery or VATS.

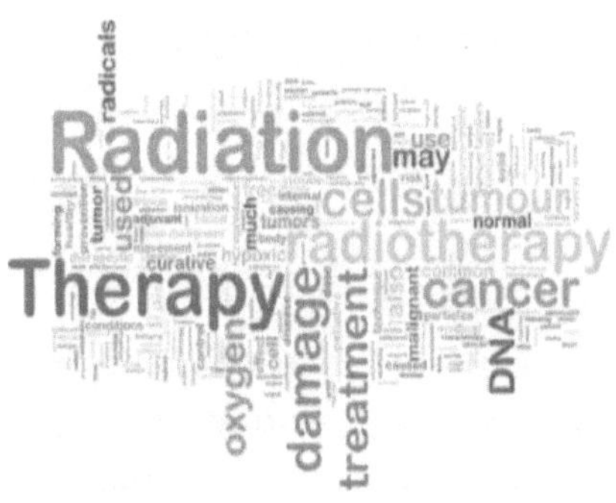

How is Lung Cancer Treated Using Radiotherapy?

More than 15% of all cancer diagnoses each year can be attributes to lung cancer. Although the signs and symptoms of lung cancer are often not noticeable early on, this type of cancer is very common. Quicker diagnosis leads to more effective treatment, which allows for an increased survival rate. Choosing the right treatment options is essential, but there are many different options to choose from.

What Factors Matter Most?

When trying to determine the best treatment option for a lung cancer patient, there are a few factors that are incredibly important. This means that the type of lung cancer must be determined including the distinguishing small-cell lung cancer from non-small-cell lung cancer. The size of the tumor has to be taken into consideration as well as the location of the growth on the lung. It is also impossible to determine the ideal treatment options without knowing if lung cancer has spread to other areas of the body.

Staging is Critical

Getting access to all of this pertinent information is critical and known as staging. Staging the type of lung cancer allows for a better understanding of the cancer type and a more effective treatment option to be chosen. Knowing if radiotherapy is the best course of treatment is almost impossible if staging of the lung cancer is not known. Staging is learned through a closer examination of eth cancer through a CT scan and biopsy of the lung. By knowing the staging of eth cancer, it is possible to predict how patent will react to treatment over time and if the cancer will eventually return.

Radiotherapy as a Lung Cancer Treatment Option

Radiotherapy is one of the most common types of treatment for lung cancer and can be used to treat a variety of lung cancer types in many different stages. It involves using high dose x-rays to kill cancer cells or to make these cancer growths smaller in size. In some cases, radiotherapy is used in combination with surgical treatments to kill all remaining cancer cells after surgery. It is possible for radiotherapy to be directed at the exact location where the cancer has spread. This means that high dose x-rays can be directed right at the lung that is affected. Although it kills all the cancerous cells, it also kills all the good cells. The effectiveness of this treatment option depends on the staging of the lung cancer.

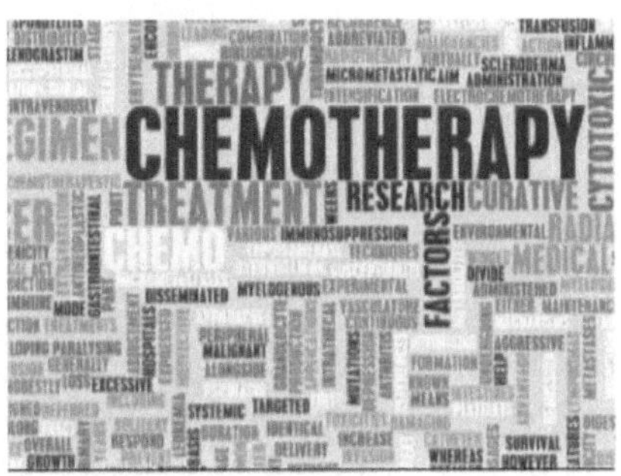

How is Lung Cancer Treated Using Chemotherapy?

Lung cancer can vary based on size and location of the growth. This means that determining the size, type and exact location of the tumor is critical to choosing the right treatment option. Lung cancer is one of the most common types of cancer and is greatly attributed to smoking, but early diagnosis of it is not always possible. Many of the signs and symptoms of lung cancer are difficult to notice and are often misdiagnosed. This means that at the first sign of symptoms, it is essential to have a doctor perform an examination and run further tests to see if lung cancer exists.

Why Does Staging Matter?

Before the right treatment option can be chosen, it is essential that staging of the lung cancer is determined. This allows for a better understanding of eth lung cancer and a prediction of how the patient will fare over time. It is also important for staging to be done to ensure if cancer has a chance of coming back depending on the course of treatment chosen.

How Does Staging Occur?

The only way to determine the staging of lung cancer is to run tests designed to further examine the progression of eth cancer. This means that CT scans and a lung biopsy are required to find out what stage of cancer before the most effective treatment can be chosen.

Is Chemotherapy a Treatment Option for Lung Cancer?

Chemotherapy is a treatment option for lung cancer and it involves the use of cytotoxic medications to kill cancer. These cytotoxic medications are designed to be cell-killing, which makes it an effective treatment option.

How Does Chemotherapy Work?

This type of treatment works within the body by killing and dividing cells. Different types of chemotherapy medications work slightly different and are designed for lung cancer in various stages. Some medications are even given in combination with others for the most effective treatment. Side effects including hair loss, nausea and low blood cell counts are common with chemotherapy.

When Is Chemotherapy Used?

This type of treatment for lung cancer is most used when the cancer has spread to other regions of eth body. This is a type of systemic treatment, which means that it can kill cancer growing in any part of eth body. This is normally the course of treatment when the lung cancer is more aggressive.

How Can Lung Cancer Be Prevented?

Lung cancer is not only the most common type of cancer in the United States, but it is also one of the most fatal. Even though there are a variety of treatment options for individuals diagnosed with lung cancer, the rate of survival is not high. Many of the treatments that are commonly used to treat other cancers including surgery, chemotherapy and radiotherapy, simply are not as effective in treating lung cancer. This means that more attention needs to be paid to preventing lung cancer instead of simply finding ways to treat it.

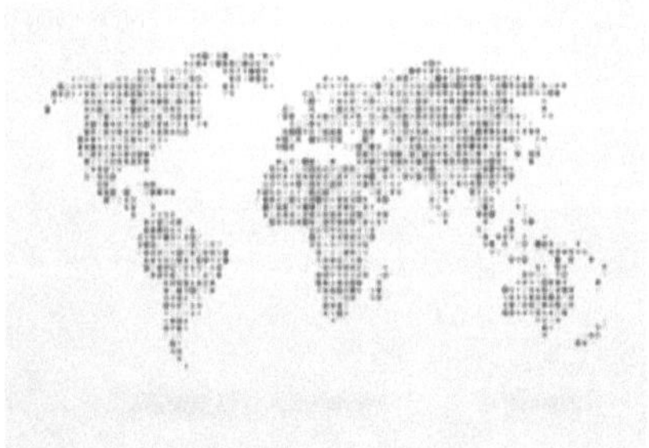

The Statistics

The fact is that most individuals with lung cancer are not diagnosed at an early stage. Tumors within the lungs can grow for years before they are noticed. This means that lung cancer prevention is even more essential since prognosis is so poor. About 60% of the people diagnosed with lung cancer die within 1 year or less and nearly 80% will die within 2 years. Even though lung cancer treatments are improving slightly, it is time to focus more on lung cancer prevention.

Can Lung Cancer Be Prevented?

Preventing lung cancer entirely is not possible, but it is possible to lower risk factors that are associated with this type of cancer. Nearly 8 out of every 10 people that are diagnosed with lung cancer are smokers. Not smoking is the simplest way to help prevent lung cancer and quitting smoking is also a viable option. No matter what age you are, it is possible to lower your risk of getting lung cancer by quitting smoking. Even though quitting smoking lowers your risk, it is always best to never start smoking in the first place. Smoking isn't the only cause of lung cancer and simply smoking does not necessarily mean you will get it, but it will put you more at risk.

What about Diet and Lung Cancer Prevention?

Focusing on your diet can be a preventative way to stay on top of your health and help prevent against lung cancer. Research shows that a diet full of certain vegetables and fruits can be effective in lessening your chance of getting lung cancer. Preventing against lung cancer entirely is not possible, but simply not smoking and making health a priority can help lower your risk. Since this diagnosis is so grim, looking for preventive ways to treat lung cancer is best.

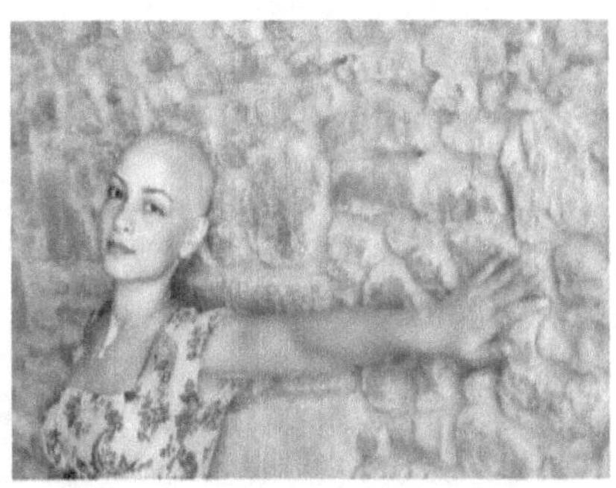

Dealing with Lung Cancer

Being diagnosed with any type of cancer can be a devastating experience from a physical and emotional standpoint. However, lung cancer is one of the most fatal types of cancer and leads to increased worry and mental decline. Dealing with lung cancer from a mental health standpoint is just as important as the treatment that is used to fight against the cancer. Once you learn that you are diagnosed with lung cancer, you will be dealing with a variety of emotions that might be difficult to control. Knowing that others are dealing with the same diagnosis as you can give you strength and hope along the way.

Shock and Denial

Many people that are diagnosed with lung cancer feel shock and denial at first. This is due to the fact that lung cancer can progress for years without you even realizing a tumor is growing. This means that you can have lung cancer that has spread to other areas of the body before you are even diagnosed. The low survival rate attached to this type of cancer also adds to eth shock and fear that many patients face initially.

Dealing with Anger

As patients begin to deal with their reality and seek treatment for their lung cancer, it is easy for anger to begin to take over. The best way to deal with the anger that you feel is to talk to a professional. Simply allowing your feelings to be released will be helpful and improve your mental health. Bottling up your anger and frustrations with your diagnosis will not help you to move forward.

Lung cancer is a unique type of cancer to deal with from an emotional standpoint, because many patients feel guilt. Almost 8 out of every 10 individuals diagnosed with lung cancer are smokers, which means that a sense of responsibility can be overwhelming. Many people with lung cancer feel guilty for continuing to smoke even though the risks are known. However, not all individuals trying to cope with lung cancer are former smokers.

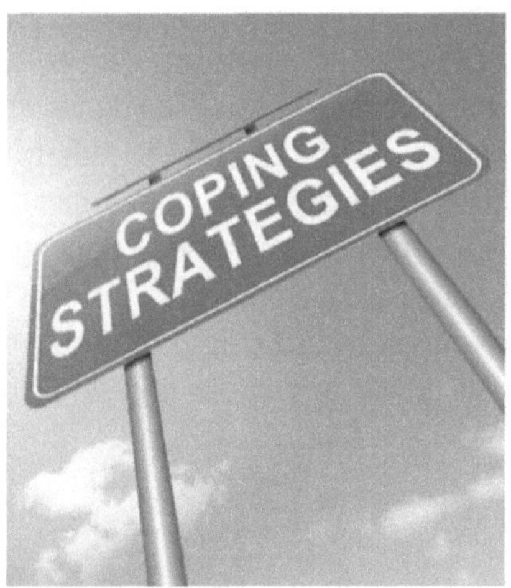

Trying to Cope

Dealing with lung cancer is not always easy emotionally, but you need to allow yourself to feel. Fear and sadness are normal and should not be feelings that are pushed away. Joining a support group of seeking professional help for coping with lung cancer will be the best way to deal with the wide range of emotions that you feel.

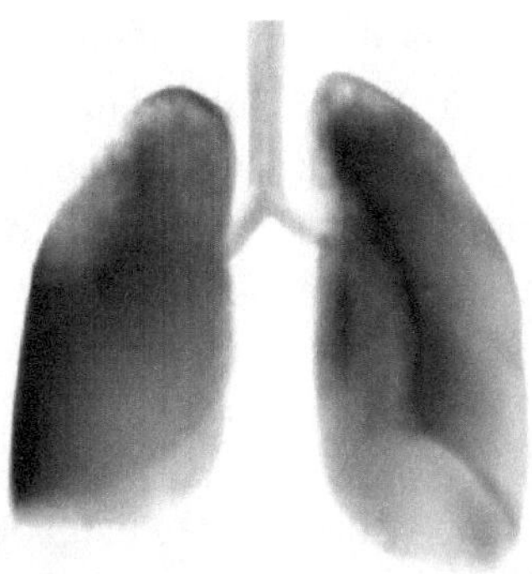

Worldwide Death Rates Attributed to Lung Cancer

Lung cancer is one of the most common types of cancer in the United States and it is very common worldwide. Even though it is so common, it is one of the most deadly forms of cancer and does not have a high survival rate. Being diagnosed with lung cancer is seen by many to be a death sentence, but there are effective treatment options that can get rid of lung cancer altogether.

What is Lung Cancer?

Lung cancer is a type of cancer that involves the growth of abnormal cells within the lungs. These abnormal cells can result in a tumor that inhibits the shape and function of the lung. The reason that the death rate for lung cancer is so high worldwide, is due to the lack of early diagnosis. Most cases of lung cancer are not noticed or diagnosed right away, which is the biggest factor in the high death rate. About 6 out of every 10 people diagnosed with lung cancer worldwide will die within 1 year and about 8 in 10 will die with 2 years. This means that early diagnosis is the key to lowering the death rate for lung cancer.

Treatment options and Death Rate

The fact is that common cancer treatment options are not as effective when treating lung cancer. Even though staging the cancer does have an impact on death rate, the treatment option that is best for treating lung cancer depends on the type and extent of your condition. This means that before a doctor comes up with an available treatment option, the type, size and location of the tumor need to be known. It is also important to know if the cancer has spread to any other region of the body. When cancer has spread to other parts of the body, the death rate increases.

Staging and Death Rate

The stage of lung cancer that you are diagnosed with has a big part to play in the survival rate that you can expect. Staging allows for your doctor to better predict how your cancer will progress over time and the chances that it might return. Lower stages generally are linked to a better prognosis and a treatment option that is less severe. Being diagnosed with a lower stage of lung cancer offers a higher rate of survival and a better likelihood of finding the most effective treatment option.